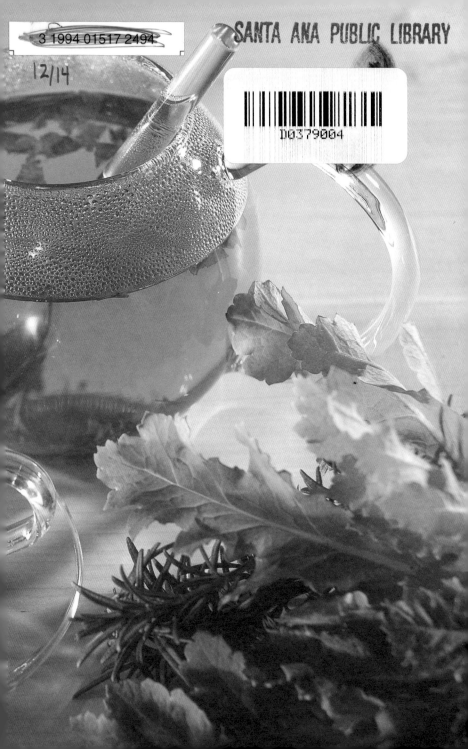

50 NATURAL WAYS TO
RELIEVE A COLD

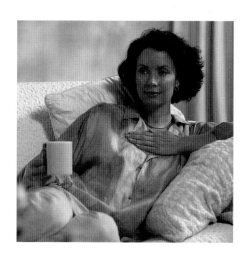

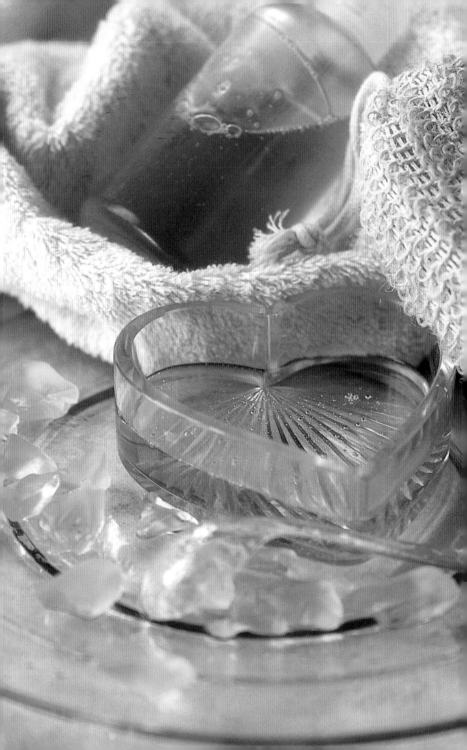

50 NATURAL WAYS TO
RELIEVE A COLD

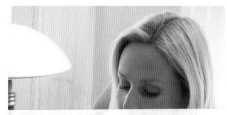

**Instant, simple hints and tips
for curing the common cold**

Raje Airey

LORENZ BOOKS

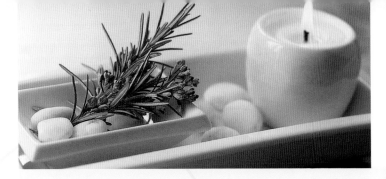

contents

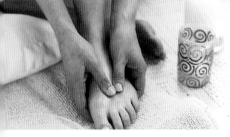

50 natural ways to...

relieve a cold

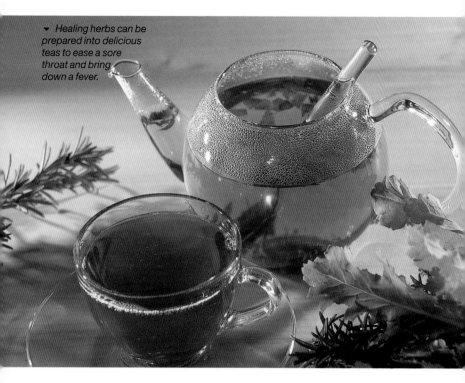

Healing herbs can be prepared into delicious teas to ease a sore throat and bring down a fever.

introduction

A cold is reputedly the most common infection that you are likely to suffer. With over 200 strains of cold virus and new flu-strains cropping up every winter, huge numbers of the population can expect to "go down" with a cold or flu-like symptoms at least once or twice a year.

With so many different cold viruses, it is perhaps not surprising that a miracle cure has not been found. Instead, a plethora of over-the-counter preparations exist to help you cope with the unpleasant symptoms of colds and flu. Generally, these treatments are based on suppressing the body's symptoms,

"knocking them on the head" so that you can carry on with your life as normal. One of the problems with many pharmaceutical drug-based products however, is that they often have undesirable side effects, which can create a new set of problems for the body. In the long term, they may even have a weakening effect on the immune system as it copes with the toxic residue from chemically produced compounds. This has encouraged a growing interest in traditional natural remedies, safely practised for hundreds of years, as people look for effective treatments that are gentle and non-toxic.

what is a cold?

The common cold is a viral infection affecting the upper respiratory system: the nose, throat and sinus passages. Every day, the air that you breathe contains many harmful viruses (pathogens), which the respiratory tract works hard to combat, fighting them off before they enter the body.

One of the body's first lines of defence is the nose: you rely on it to trap and neutralize pathogens. With central heating and a lack of fresh air, the mucous membranes of the nose and sinuses become swollen and congested with a thick secretion. When the respiratory system cannot deal with the pathogens effectively, they enter the body tissue where they begin to damage cells, causing inflammation and all the other cold-like symptoms.

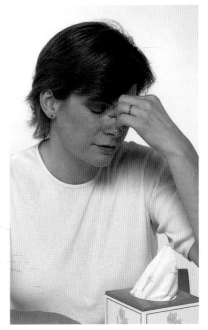

▲ A blocked-up nose is the perfect breeding ground for germs.

general symptoms

Colds usually come on suddenly and the symptoms are relatively mild and of limited duration, lasting on average a week to ten days. Typically, the first stage of a cold is characterized by sneezing, watery eyes and a sore throat as the mucous membranes become inflamed. This may be accompanied by shivering and feeling chilly, usually a sign of a raised temperature as the body attempts to kill off the invading germs. Other signs of a raised temperature include aching limbs and feeling weak, as the viruses spread beyond the primary site of infection (in the nose and throat), into the blood and on to different organs and tissues in the body. The body then becomes vulnerable to secondary respiratory infections such as sinusitis, laryngitis, ear infections and bronchitis, which are usually more unpleasant and much more serious than the original cold.

During a cold the body produces more mucus in order to help trap the invading germs. Once the drippy, runny nose stage dries up, it can turn into a blocked, stuffed-up head cold, which may also be accompanied by a cough.

coughs

A cough is a reflex action of the bronchi, designed to clear the airways of excessive mucus. Coughs can be divided into two types, each needing different treatments. A loose, moist "productive" cough needs remedies that help the body to expel the excess mucus. With a dry, tickling cough, the mucous membranes have become so inflamed that they provoke coughing even when there is no mucus to clear. This type of cough can be exhausting and calls for treatments that soothe the inflammation and help to reduce aggravating bronchial spasm.

catching a cold

The common-sense belief is that colds are created through catching a germ. Although this statement is partly true, it doesn't explain why some people catch colds and others, even if they have been exposed to the same virus, do not. First, you have to create a suitable breeding ground in the body before a germ can take hold. When you catch a cold, it means that your immune system is below par in some way and your body is unable to fight off infection. There are various reasons why this may be so, and there are many things that you can do to try to prevent this happening.

lifestyle indicators

Research indicates that many respiratory problems originate in an unhealthy lifestyle. Lack of fresh air and exercise, shallow breathing, poor posture, smoking and air pollution all place a strain on the lungs. Similarly, eating a diet high in dairy produce, sugar and refined carbohydrates places a strain on the body, as these foods weaken the immune system

and encourage the build-up of mucus. Good health is linked with a balanced lifestyle. Regular exercise, sufficient rest and sleep, a balanced diet, satisfying work and fulfilling relationships all contribute towards health and wellbeing.

When any area of life is out of balance, it places a strain on the immune system. The greater the duration and level of stress, the more the immune system is weakened. You can encourage the immune system to stay strong and healthy by drinking more fresh juices and mineral water, and eating plenty of organic fruit, vegetables and salad.

holistic medicine

In natural medicine, a cold is not necessarily seen as a bad thing as it may be the body's way of trying to clear out toxins from the system and of giving the body a much-needed rest. Consequently, natural treatments are not based on ignoring and/or suppressing a cold, but are designed to work with the body, recognizing its symptoms as part of the body's self-healing process.

Holistic medicine is about finding ways to encourage your body to stay strong and healthy, and using drug-free treatments, free from side effects, whenever you do become sick.

Whether you are suffering from a runny nose, a sore throat, aching limbs, a raised temperature or blocked sinuses, this book is packed with a variety of non-pharmaceutical remedies to help alleviate your symptoms.

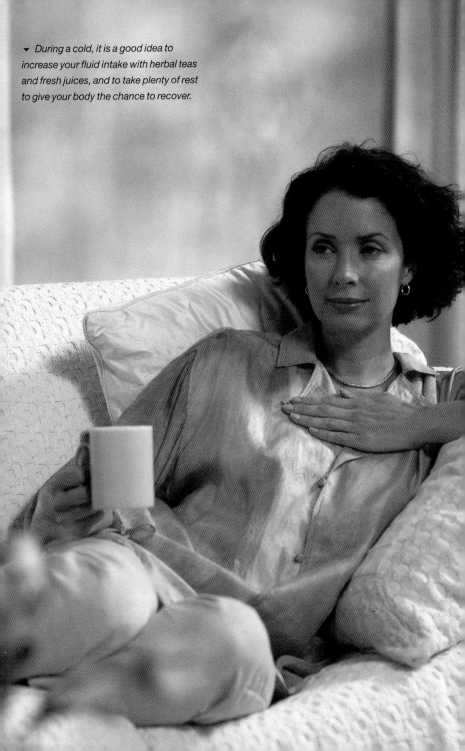

During a cold, it is a good idea to increase your fluid intake with herbal teas and fresh juices, and to take plenty of rest to give your body the chance to recover.

cold treatments

There are literally hundreds of natural remedies that can heal and soothe a cold and strengthen the immune system. The following pages contain 50 of the most effective methods, many of which have been tried and tested for centuries and used in different healing traditions across the world. All the treatments are based on holistic principles – where the pathway to health is seen as a fine balance between mental, physical and emotional wellbeing – and are designed to stimulate the body's own healing ability. They include energy therapies, such as homeopathy, reiki and crystal healing, as well as hands-on methods, such as massage and reflexology. There are also treatments based on nutrition, vitamins, minerals and medicinal foods, together with many herbal remedies, utilizing a plant's leaves, fruits and flowers to make gargles, teas, cordials, syrups, lotions and tonics. With 50 natural treatments to choose from, you're bound to find the remedy to suit your needs.

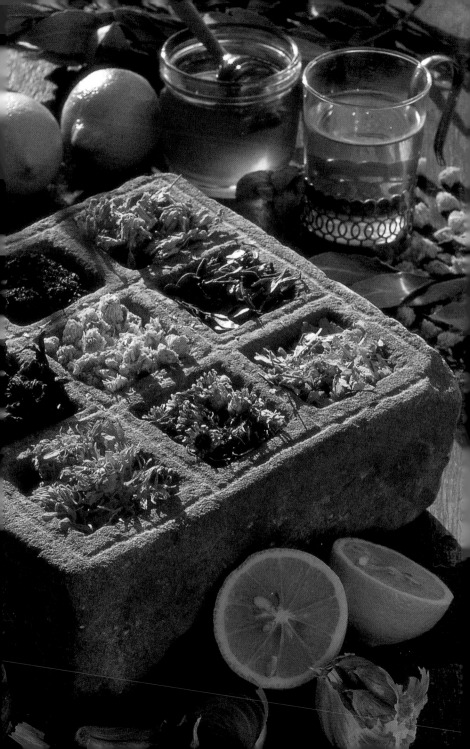

1

strengthening vitamin C

A strong immune system is vital for good health. Vitamin C plays an essential role in supporting the immune system to fight infection, and has potent antiviral and antibacterial properties.

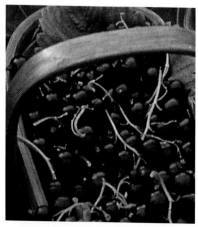

▲ Fresh blackcurrants are a good source of vitamin C. Eat them lightly cooked or raw.

to one 1000mg dose taken once a day, then to 500mg a day as a maintenance dose to keep coughs and colds at bay. Therapeutic doses of vitamin C are best taken as a dietary supplement in the form of tablets or effervescent powders.

The best natural sources of vitamin C are found in fruit and vegetables, particularly citrus fruits, blackcurrants, berries, rosehips, peppers, green leafy vegetables, carrots and sweet potatoes. It is best to consume these foods raw (except for rosehips and potatoes), as vitamin C is destroyed by cooking.

Vitamin C is used up more rapidly under stress and when fighting colds or infection. The body is unable to store or produce this water-soluble vitamin, and relies on an adequate daily intake. For this reason, vitamin C is generally regarded as safe to take in therapeutic doses, as any excess is excreted via the kidneys.

For treating colds, many health care practitioners recommend a therapeutic dose of 1000mg taken three times a day. This should be gradually reduced

BEST FOOD SOURCES OF VITAMIN C
IN MG PER 100G

Rosehip syrup	295
Blackcurrants	200
Guavas	200
Parsley	150
Broccoli	110
Green peppers	100
Citrus fruits	50-80
Watercress	60
All other fruit and vegetables	20-40

2

essential zinc

Lowered zinc levels impair the healthy functioning of the immune system. If you feel run down, suffer frequent colds and have a poor sense of taste or smell, it could be that you are deficient in zinc.

Zinc is an essential mineral that is involved in many bodily processes and is necessary for normal cell division and function. Unfortunately research indicates that zinc deficiencies are fairly common in large numbers of the population. The body's reserves of zinc are depleted by stress, vigorous exercise (the mineral is lost through excessive sweating), smoking, and high intakes of tea, coffee, alcohol and refined foods. Even if you eat plenty of fresh fruit and vegetables, they are likely to have been grown in soils that are low in vital minerals and trace elements, including zinc.

Some of the best natural sources of zinc are found in shellfish, particularly oysters, crabs and mussels. Liver and dried brewer's yeast are also high in zinc, and other sources include hard cheese, eggs, beef, turkey and pumpkin seeds.

To make sure you are getting enough zinc, take a zinc supplement of between 15-20mg a day with a

glass of orange juice (vitamin C aids zinc absorption). Zinc supplements should not be taken on an empty stomach as they may cause nausea.

For a cold, you could try sucking zinc lozenges, which are available in good health stores and pharmacies. It seems that the mineral may have a direct action on the cold viruses in the mouth, nose and throat, which stops them multiplying.

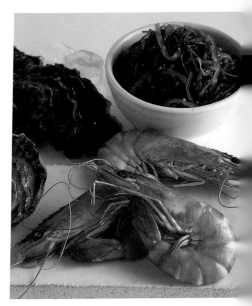

▸ *Making shellfish a regular part of your diet will help to increase your zinc levels.*

3 potent echinacea

During the last 50 years, echinacea has become increasingly famous for its healing properties. It is a powerful immunity booster and helps the body deal with bacterial and viral infections.

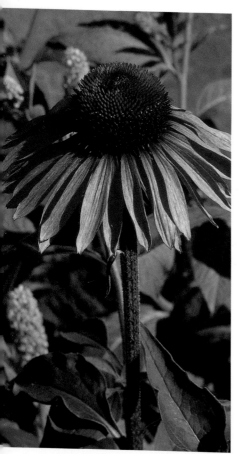

▲ *Today, echinacea is regarded as one of the world's foremost medicinal herbs.*

The Native Americans have used echinacea for hundreds of years to treat all kinds of illnesses, including poisonous bites, stubborn wounds and fevers. Research indicates that echinacea is an effective antibiotic, with powerful antiviral, antifungal and antibacterial properties. It is particularly useful for warding off upper respiratory infections.

Echinacea tincture is available in good health stores and pharmacies. To treat colds and infections of the upper respiratory tract, take 2.5ml/½ tsp of tincture in a glass of mineral water or fresh orange juice, two or three times a day. As a preventative measure, take 2.5ml/½ tsp as before, once a day. If you prefer, echinacea is also available in capsule or tablet form. For colds, take a 500mg capsule three times a day.

Because of its effective action on the immune system, echinacea is being investigated as a possible treatment for HIV and AIDS. It is useful for treating chronic infections, as well as day-to-day coughs, colds and catarrh.

4 antiseptic garlic

King of all healing plants, garlic is one of nature's "swear by" remedies. This powerful antiseptic was regularly used to treat all kinds of infections before the development of antibiotics.

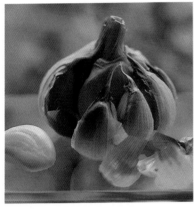

▲ An average clove of garlic contains substances equivalent to roughly one-fifth of an average penicillin dose.

To get the most from garlic's health-giving properties, get into the habit of adding a little to your daily diet − it will help keep you strong and healthy.

Raw garlic is best, but one of the problems with garlic is its pungent odour and taste, which is not to everyone's liking. Eating fresh parsley or tarragon helps to reduce garlic breath, and lightly stir-frying the cloves for a few moments also helps to eliminate any unpleasant after-effects. The cloves can be crushed, chopped or left whole, with crushed garlic having the strongest flavour. When cooking, make sure that the garlic does not turn brown as this will make it taste bitter. Add the garlic to food prior to serving.

To treat a cold, you should eat up to six fresh cloves a day. If you cannot bear the taste or smell, odourless garlic capsules are widely available from health food stores as well as most supermarkets. You should take 1-3 garlic capsules daily.

• Garlic has antibacterial and antiviral properties and a long tradition of medicinal use. Slaves in ancient Egypt were fed it to keep them strong, traditional Chinese herbalists prescribed it, chewed raw, to keep coughs and colds at bay, and both ancient Greek and Roman physicians prescribed garlic to treat respiratory infections.

• A quick and easy way of using garlic is to rub the inside of a salad bowl with a clove of raw garlic before adding the salad leaves.

5 healthy eating

Hippocrates is credited with saying "let food be thy medicine and medicine be thy food". Support the immune system to stay strong and eat a healthy diet – it will increase the body's resistance to colds.

Food provides the body with the raw materials it needs to function effectively. A healthy diet is one that contains plenty of fresh fruit and vegetables, salads, wholegrains, nuts and seeds. If you eat meat and/or fish, include a little chicken, turkey, game, lean red meat, shellfish and oily fish such as salmon, mackerel, herrings and tuna. Meat-eaters and vegetarians alike should include soya bean products, such as tofu or tempeh. Soya is a perfect source of protein, and research suggests that it offers protection against certain diseases.

Include generous amounts of raw food in your diet as all forms of cooking reduce some of the nutritional qualities of the raw ingredients. Some practitioners recommend that one

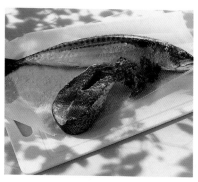

▲ *Eat oily fish such as mackerel or salmon.*

third of your daily food intake should be raw. When cooking, lightly stir-fried food is preferable to baked or fried.

Choose organic food whenever possible. It is produced without the use of chemical pesticides and fertilizers, some of which are highly toxic.

healthy eating tips

For snacking, eat 2-3 pieces of fresh fruit a day, or keep a store of nuts and raisins. Remember to increase your water intake to 2 litres/3½ pints a day. This will help rid your system of toxins.

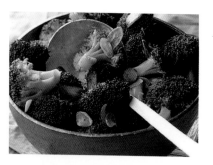

◄ *Dark green vegetables, such as broccoli, form part of a healthy eating regime.*

6 easy breathing

Every year, more and more people are suffering from respiratory disorders, including colds, congested sinuses and chronic catarrh. These problems can be made worse by certain foods.

During a cold or respiratory infection, avoid sugar, cheese and dairy products, and processed, refined foods. This means saying "no" to white bread, pasta, cakes, pizza, any fast-food, and many commercial preparations, which tend to be highly processed and very often contain sugar. All of these foods encourage the production of mucus, which adds to the congestion in an overloaded respiratory system.

Tea, coffee, fizzy drinks and alcohol are also best avoided as they have a weakening effect on the immune system. Try fresh juices, herbal teas and plenty of mineral water instead.

easy breathing tips

To keep the lungs and airways healthy, eat plenty of unrefined, unprocessed foods. Additionally there are certain foods that seem to have a protective action on the respiratory system. Green vegetables, such as broccoli, peas, spinach and watercress are a good source of immunity boosting antioxidants. Carrots, sweet potatoes, apricots and mangoes are all high in betacarotene, from which the body can obtain vitamin A, which is

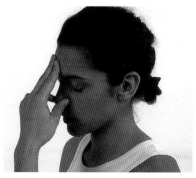

▲ Blocked sinuses are made worse by eating fast foods, dairy products and sugar.

anti-infective and supports the mucus membranes. Eating plenty of citrus fruits, rich in vitamin C, together with onions, garlic, ginger and chilli will all help to open the airways and clear out mucus.

During a cold, avoid mucus-forming foods (these include dairy products and refined carbohydrates) and maintain a regular intake of garlic, ideally fresh. Garlic not only helps to stimulate the removal of excess mucus, but is one of the most powerful anti-infective agents available.

7 carrot revitalizer

Nutritious and easy to prepare, home-made juices are 100% pure, with nothing added or taken away. They are packed with essential vitamins and minerals and are excellent immunity boosters.

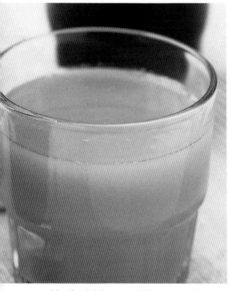

▲ *Use fresh juices straight away, as they lose their potency if they are left standing.*

Fresh carrots are one of nature's wonderfoods and are ideal for juicing. They are easy to obtain all the year round and are packed with vitamins. A single carrot is so rich in betacarotene that it provides an adequate daily intake of vitamin A, the vitamin that is necessary to maintain resistance against respiratory infections. It is also high in vitamins C and E, with vitamin E also protecting the lungs against pollution and respiratory infections.

carrot, apple and orange juice
Carrot juice has a mild sweet taste, which mixes well with other fruit and vegetable juices. Try it with orange and apple juice, both fruits that are high in vitamin C. To make enough for one serving, take three carrots, scrubbed and trimmed, one apple, washed and cut into quarters, and an orange which has been peeled and cut into segments. Using a juice extractor, juice the carrots and fruit and pour into a glass. Serve immediately and drink by sipping slowly.

Make fresh fruit and vegetable juices a regular part of your healthy eating plan. They support the immune system, are easy to digest, and help keep the body clean and free of toxins. They are packed with energy and healing properties – and they taste good too.

Squeeze citrus fruits
and drink the
juice neat or
diluted with water to ward off
a cold and ease a
sore throat.

9 stimulating ginger

Ginger is widely used in traditional Chinese medicine to treat chills, fever, headaches and aching muscles, and the early European herbalists also recognized it as a cure for colds.

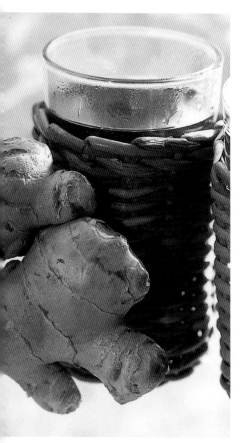

Ginger is a powerful immunity booster whose antiseptic, warming, anti-inflammatory and invigorating properties make it an invaluable medicine for the treatment of colds. This fiery spice stimulates the circulation and restores vitality, promoting feelings of wellbeing. It is especially useful during the long, cold, damp months of winter.

immunity-boosting lunch
Always make sure you have a supply of fresh ginger root available in the kitchen and get into the habit of using it in your cooking. A little fresh ginger root is delicious grated into a raw carrot salad. Try it for an immunity-boosting lunch – it will give you lots of energy for the afternoon.

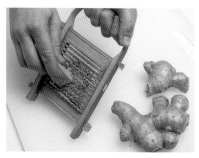

▲ ▶ *Ginger encourages the body to eliminate toxins, it opens up the nasal passages and has an expectorant action on the lungs.*

10 warming cayenne

The scarlet fruit pods (chillies) of the cayenne pepper plant have medicinal and culinary uses. The pods may be used whole or crushed to make powder, and are antibacterial and rich in vitamin C.

The heat of cayenne makes it useful as a strengthening tonic for the immune system and for warding off winter blues, lethargy and chills. Both the pods and the powder are powerful stimulants, boosting poor circulation and bringing warmth and vitality to the whole body. In particular, cayenne is excellent for treating the respiratory system. It is a powerful decongestant and expectorant and its pungency encourages the airways to open up, helping to alleviate the symptoms of a stuffy cold.

For general good health, try adding fresh chillies or cayenne powder to soups, curries and stews. To treat a cold or sore throat, add a pinch of cayenne powder to lemon juice, dilute with hot water and sweeten with honey. Drink three times daily.

CAUTIONS

• Extract the seeds from fresh chillies as these can be toxic.

• Avoid therapeutic doses of cayenne during pregnancy and while you are breastfeeding.

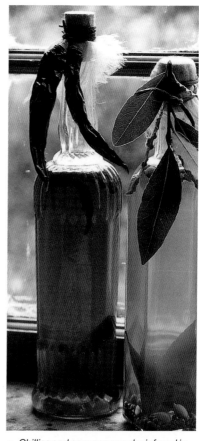

▲ Chillies and cayenne powder infused in cider vinegar make an effective medicine for treating the symptoms of a cold.

11 comforting cinnamon

For thousands of years, cinnamon has been used in the treatment of colds and flu. It warms and energizes the body, helping to ward off infection, and combat the listless feeling so typical of flu.

Cinnamon is a potent antiseptic, tonic and stimulant, which possesses antispasmodic properties. This sweetly pungent spice is taken from the inner bark of the cinnamon tree and is available as a brownish powder, or as small, delicately rolled sticks.

The bark of cinnamon promotes sweating and is ideal for treating "cold" conditions in the body, helping to relieve the aches and chills in the early stages of a cold or flu. Cinnamon sticks are often added to fruit punches in the winter for their warm, spicy aroma and their comforting effect.

The distinctive flavour and aroma of cinnamon combines well with oranges, which are rich in vitamin C. To make yourself a delicious hot toddy, add a stick of cinnamon to a glass of freshly squeezed orange juice. Top up with hot water and sweeten with honey. This health-giving drink should help to beat the winter blues and fight off infection.

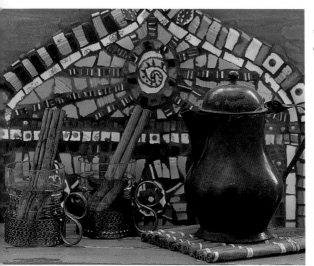

◄ *A hot orange tea flavoured with cinnamon makes a delicious drink to treat a cold.*

A centrally heated atmosphere can be a breeding ground for germs. Make sure you have enough fresh air and exercise to help the immune system stay strong.

12 soothing liquorice

Liquorice root has a cooling, soothing effect on mucus membranes. Its antispasmodic and expectorant action helps the airways to open up and expel or disperse any phlegm.

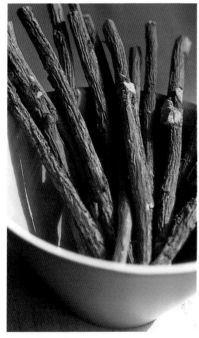

▲ *Liquorice root is traditionally used to treat a wide range of respiratory problems.*

In ancient Greece, liquorice was taken for asthma, chest problems and mouth ulcers – often a sign of being run down. Liquorice contains a substance 50 times sweeter than sugar, which stimulates the adrenals and encourages the body to produce its own hydrocortisone. In modern medicine, hydrocortisone is an important drug that is used to treat serious inflammatory conditions, including chronic chest problems.

liquorice cough tea

Dried liquorice root is generally available in good health stores. This can be boiled up in the proportion of 115g/4oz piece of dried liquorice root to 600ml/1 pint/2½ cups water to make a soothing tea. Alternatively, a few unsweetened black liquorice sticks can be covered in boiling water and left to dissolve. This will produce a strong extract that can be used to ease a chesty cough.

The dried, woody root of the liquorice plant is not only widely used in confectionery but has a tradition of medicinal use stretching back thousands of years. In Chinese medicine, liquorice is known as the "great detoxifier" as it is thought to drive poisons from the system.

13 elderflower tisane

Increasing fluid intake during a cold helps the body decongest and eliminate toxins. Tea, coffee and caffeinated drinks are best avoided and can be substituted with herb and spice teas instead.

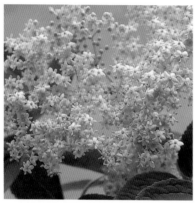

◀ *Elderflowers have been valued for their medicinal uses for thousands of years.*

Although you can buy herbal teas ready-made, making them fresh increases their health-giving properties. An easy way of making herbal teas is as an infusion or tisane, when the fresh or dried leaves, stems or flowers of a plant are left to steep in near-boiling water, which is then strained off and drunk.

A tisane of elderflower, chamomile and peppermint will help relieve many symptoms of a feverish cold. Peppermint has cooling properties and a stimulating, decongestant action. This is attributed to its high menthol content, making it particularly effective for clearing blocked sinuses and a stuffy nose. Elderflowers have anticatarrhal properties and encourage sweating, helping a fever to "come out", while chamomile flowers have a gentle anti-inflammatory, antispasmodic action and are a natural sedative. They are useful for bringing a fever down, soothing a racking and persistent cough, and promoting rest and sleep.

elderflower cold cure

To make the tea, the fresh or dried plant constituents may be used. You will need 2.5ml/½ tsp of each herb per 250ml/8fl oz/1 cup of near-boiling water. For fresh flowers and leaves, double up the quantities of each herb. Add the herbs to the hot water and leave to infuse for 5–10 minutes. Strain the liquid off and gently reheat if necessary. Pour into a mug and add a slice of lemon and a little honey to sweeten. For an extra warming effect, add a sprinkling of ground ginger. Drink the tea two or three times a day to combat a cold.

14 horehound infusion

Herbal teas are warm and comforting to drink and can help to ward off coughs and colds. They also bring relief from unpleasant symptoms – horehound can ease a feverish cold and a chesty cough.

The bitter juice extracted from the flowers and leaves of white horehound is an expectorant and a soothing tonic for the mucus membranes, making it a traditional cough medicine ingredient. Horehound is also a mild stimulant; it can relieve the groggy feeling that accompanies a bad cold.

horehound cough tea

Add some chopped fresh or dried leaves to 250ml/8fl oz/1 cup of near-boiling water. Infuse for 15 minutes, and strain off the liquid. Sweeten to taste with a little honey. This mixture may be drunk as a tea, three times daily between meals, or used as a gargle to alleviate a sore throat.

▾ *Use horehound to ease a hacking cough.*

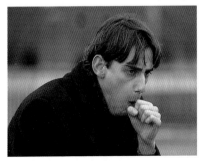

As well as being made into an infusion for drinking and gargling, horehound extract may be added to sugar syrup and boiled down to make cough candy.

▾ *Drinking herbal teas is a good way to look after yourself when you have a cold.*

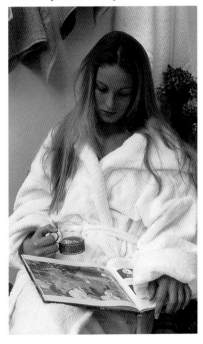

15 thyme infusion

In herbal medicine, thyme is recognized for its antiseptic properties and for its special affinity with the respiratory system. This makes it a valuable remedy for treating coughs and colds.

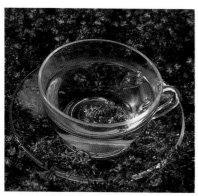

▲ An infusion made from thyme has a pungent taste, and its warming properties are good for treating chills.

thyme cold treatment tea

Both the leaves and pink flowering tops can be used to make an infusion. For a brew, use 5ml/1 tsp dried thyme, or 10ml/2 tsp fresh, per 250ml/ 8fl oz/1 cup of near-boiling water. Steep the herbs in the water for 10 minutes, then drain off the liquid into a cup. Sweeten with honey if desired, add a slice of lemon and drink while hot. Drink the tea three times a day between meals.

Thyme contains the volatile oil, thymol, which has strong antiseptic, antifungal and antibacterial properties. These antiseptic properties make thyme a useful tonic for the immune system, as well as an effective remedy for chesty coughs and colds. Thyme has a powerful action on the respiratory system, producing expectoration and reducing bronchial spasm. It also has a warming, calming effect on the body and is useful during the chilly, shivering stage of a cold.

▼ Relaxing quietly and keeping warm will help a cold clear up more quickly.

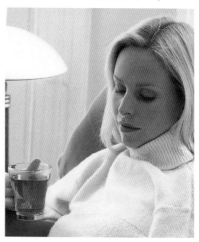

16 sage, honey & lemon tea

A sore throat is often one of the first signs of a cold. Sage has powerful antiseptic, antibiotic and astringent properties and is useful for treating infections – particularly of the mouth and throat.

To ease a raspy throat, the juice of a freshly squeezed lemon combined with bitter sage leaves and sweetened with honey, produces a comforting, pleasant-tasting drink, packed with healing properties. Like sage, lemon is also a potent antiseptic and anti-inflammatory. This, together with its high vitamin C content, makes lemon a good choice for sore throats.

sage throat soother

For a soothing tea, mix together 25g/ 1oz dried sage leaves with 30ml/ 2 tbsp clear honey. Add the freshly-squeezed juice of a lemon, then dilute with 600ml/1 pint/2½ cups boiling water. Cover and leave to infuse for about 20-30 minutes. Strain into a non-aluminium pan and reheat the mixture until hot enough for drinking. Drink or gargle with the tea several times a day as needed.

CAUTIONS
- Avoid sage tea during pregnancy as it may stimulate uterine contractions.

- Thujone (an active ingredient of sage), can trigger fits in epileptics.

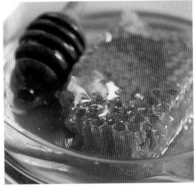

▲ Honey is also a natural antibiotic.

▼ Both lemon and sage are antiseptic.

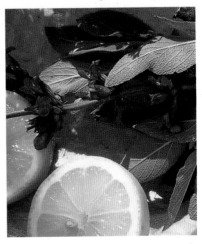

17 rosehip decoction

The high levels of vitamins and other nutrients found in rosehips are readily absorbed by the body. Rosehips should be picked when ripe and can be used fresh or dried to make delicious herbal teas.

Whole, dried rosehips will need softening and cooking in order to release their nutrients. This method of cooking herbs and spices to extract their therapeutic properties is known as decocting.

> Rosehips are good for you: a single rosehip typically contains 20 times more vitamin C than an average-sized orange.

▼ *Rosehip tea has a sweet astringent taste.*

rosehip cold cure

To make fresh rosehip tea, take 2-3 washed rosehips, top and tail them and leave them to soak overnight. Now fill a non-aluminium pan with 600ml/1 pint/2½ cups water and bring it to the boil. Add the rosehips and simmer for about 30 minutes. Finish by straining the mixture into a mug or cup, and add a little honey to sweeten if you wish. Drink the tea at intervals throughout the day – it will help the body to flush out toxins.

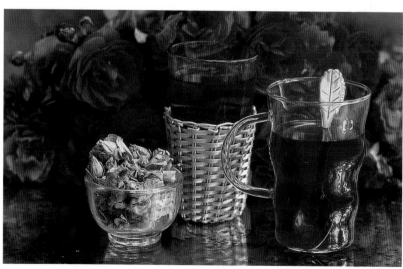

18 ginger & lemon tea

Keep ginger and lemon on standby for the onset of a shivery cold. Ginger is warming and stimulating and combines well with the sharp citrus tang of lemon to help the body fight off viral infections.

Decoctions are typically used to make medicinal concoctions from the root and bark of a plant. Ginger is extracted from the root of the ginger plant by boiling. The decoction lasts 2–3 days.

ginger and lemon decoction

To make a delicious hot ginger and lemon drink, take a 115g/4oz piece of washed fresh root ginger and slice it into 600ml/1 pint/2½ cups water in a non-aluminium pan. Take a lemon and grate it finely, adding the rind to the pan with a pinch of cayenne pepper. Bring the water to the boil, cover the pan and simmer for 20 minutes. Meanwhile, squeeze the rest of the lemon into a cup. When the ginger mixture has finished cooking, remove it from the heat and allow it to cool slightly before adding the lemon juice. Strain off the liquid, add honey to taste, and drink several times a day as needed.

Ginger stimulates the circulation, encouraging sweating, the elimination of toxins and the expulsion of mucus and catarrh.

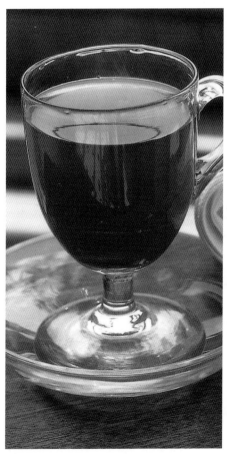

▲ *Enjoy a hot ginger and lemon toddy at bedtime – it's a traditional cold cure.*

19 hibiscus & rosehip tea

Hibiscus flowers have a soothing antispasmodic action, helpful for reducing fevers and soothing coughs. They combine well with rosehips – both plants are an excellent source of vitamin C.

Hibiscus flowers are a popular ingredient in many herbal teas. In Egypt, they form the basis of *karkade*, a chilled tea, traditionally served to travellers as a restorative after a long journey. Combined with rosehips, hibiscus makes a delicious, refreshing drink that is useful for treating cold symptoms or, better still, for keeping cold viruses at bay.

hibiscus and rosehip refresher
To make this soothing hibiscus and rosehip infusion, take two washed fresh rosehips. Top, tail and chop them up and place them in a bowl. Now add enough water to cover them, and leave to soak overnight. When the rosehip pieces are soft, strain off the water and add them to 5ml/1 tsp dried hibiscus flower petals. Add 250ml/8fl oz/ 1 cup of near-boiling water, cover and leave to infuse. When the mixture is ready, strain it into a non-aluminium pan and reheat until hot enough to drink. Pour the tea into a cup and sweeten with a little honey to taste. Drink regularly throughout the day as required.

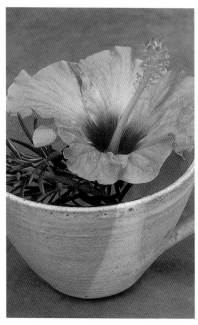

▲ *Hibiscus flowers are a delicious pick-me-up with many health-giving properties.*

CAUTION
Hibiscus *rosa-sinensis* is the medicinal variety, and should not be confused with the ornamental Hibiscus *sino-chinensis*, which is not suitable for making tea.

20 nasturtium tisane

Nasturtium is a traditional remedy of the Peruvian Indians for coughs, colds and flu. European herbalists used it to treat a wide range of ills, including scurvy and respiratory complaints.

Nasturtium was helpful against scurvy because of its high vitamin C content, and modern research shows that fresh nasturtium leaves contain a natural antibiotic that is effective in treating respiratory conditions. Nasturtium has powerful antimicrobial and decongestant properties and a warming and stimulating action on the body. This pungent and bitter plant is a good blood cleanser, stimulating the liver and helping the elimination of toxins. In order to treat respiratory congestion, some modern-day herbalists recommend eating 3 fresh nasturtium leaves a day. You can also add nasturtium flowers to a salad for a decorative and nutritious effect.

nasturtium cleanser

If you prefer, you can take nasturtium as a tea, using either the fresh or dried leaves. To make an infusion, pour a cup of near-boiling water on 10ml/ 2 tsp fresh, chopped leaves, or 5ml/ 1 tsp of the dried leaves and leave to stand for 10–15 minutes. Strain and drink three times a day to relieve colds, catarrh and chest infections.

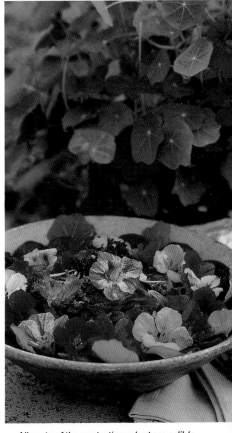

▲ All parts of the nasturtium plant are edible and nutritious; nasturtium is rich in iron, vitamin C, minerals and trace elements.

21 hyssop cold cleanser

Hyssop has been valued for thousands of years for its cleansing and purifying properties. It is a powerful antiseptic, excellent for warding off infection and strengthening the immune system.

The Cherokee Indians used the bitter leaves and delicate purple flowers of the hyssop plant to relieve respiratory disorders. Its expectorant and anticatarrhal properties, together with a general affinity for the respiratory tract, make hyssop useful for treating coughs, colds and flu, plus associated disorders such as cold sores, catarrh, sinus problems and bronchitis. Additionally, hyssop has a warming and stimulating action on the circulatory system, helping to promote sweating, bring down fevers and cleanse the blood.

▾ *The fragrant flowers of the hyssop plant are much loved by bees and butterflies.*

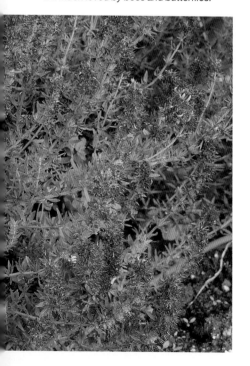

hyssop and orange tisane
The best way to take hyssop is in tea form. Add a few fresh or 5ml/1 tsp dried leaves and flowers to 250ml/ 8fl oz/1 cup of near-boiling water. Cover and leave to infuse for about 20-30 minutes. Strain into a non-aluminium pan and reheat the mixture until almost boiling. As hyssop is bitter, sweeten the tea with a little honey. For extra flavour, add a little freshly squeezed orange juice.

Hyssop has antiviral properties, and is useful for treating the herpes simplex virus, which causes cold sores. Dab a few drops of the tea on to a cotton pad at the first sign of itching.

22 lime blossom cooler

Lime blossom has a gentle, calming effect on the nervous system and is ideal for treating irritating, spasmodic coughs, soothing sore throats and bringing down a fever. Enjoy it as an infusion.

The yellow flowers of the lime or linden tree are acknowledged in folklore for their healing and restorative powers.

lime blossom tisane

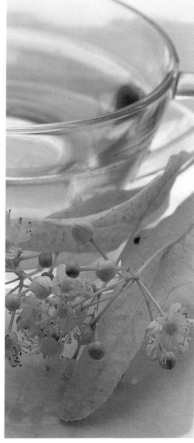

The gentle, soothing action of lime blossom makes it particularly suitable for treating children's coughs, colds and fevers. Use the weaker version of the tea (1 tsp of dried flower heads, steeped for 4 minutes) and serve three times a day.

▲ *Lime blossom tisane has a delicate, pale lemon colour and a subtle taste.*

23 elderflower & lime cordial

Fruit cordials are a pleasant way to enjoy the health-giving properties of plants. Home-made ones will keep refrigerated for several months, stored in a screw-top bottle.

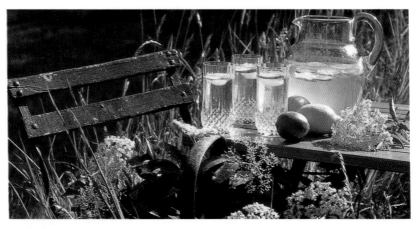

▲ *To avoid a summer cold, drink vitamin C-rich elderflower cordial.*

summer cold refresher
10 fresh elderflower heads
2–3 limes, sliced
675g/1½ lb/3 cups sugar
5ml/1 tsp citric acid
5ml/1 tsp cream of tartar
1 litre/1¾ pints/4 cups boiling water

Wash and pick over the elderflowers thoroughly, discarding any that are past their best. Put them into a large bowl with the sliced limes. Add the sugar, citric acid and cream of tartar.

Set aside for up to 12 hours. Pour in the boiling water and leave to stand for 24 hours. Strain the syrup into sterilized bottles and seal the contents with corks. To serve, dilute with about twice as much still or sparkling mineral water.

To treat a summer cold, try this deliciously refreshing elderflower and lime cordial: limes have a high vitamin C content and elderflowers are anticatarrhal. The drink is soothing on the throat and its zingy flavour will lift your spirits whenever you feel unwell. It will keep refrigerated for 2–3 months.

24 elderberry rob

Ripe elderberries are rich in vitamins A and C. They can be made into syrups and wines for preventing and treating coughs and colds, to bring down fevers and to soothe sore throats.

Elderberry is one of the oldest known medicinal herbs with expectorant and antiviral properties. Home-made elderberry cordial is easy to make and a useful standby for the winter season. The cordial can be diluted with hot or cold water and lemon juice to relieve a feverish cold and support the immune system, or taken neat as a cough and throat soother. During a cold, drink two or three glasses a day.

elderberry winter warmer
1kg/2¼ lb elderberries
350g/12oz/1½ cups sugar
grated rind and juice of an orange
10 crushed coriander seeds
1 cinnamon stick

Put all the ingredients into a non-aluminium pan and heat gently until the sugar is dissolved. Let the mixture simmer over a low heat for 20 minutes. When the liquid has cooled, strain and pour into a sterilized screw-top bottle. The cordial will keep refrigerated for several months.

▶ *Elderberries are packed with health-giving properties to ease the symptoms of a cold.*

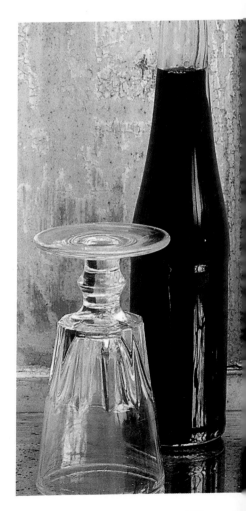

25 thyme & borage linctus

The decongestant and expectorant action of borage makes it a traditional ingredient in cough syrup recipes. It combines well with the antiseptic properties of thyme.

Making your own cough syrup is quite an easy process. The following thyme and borage linctus will keep refrigerated for up to 2 months in a screw-top bottle. Take 5ml/1 tsp as needed to ease a dry, scratchy cough.

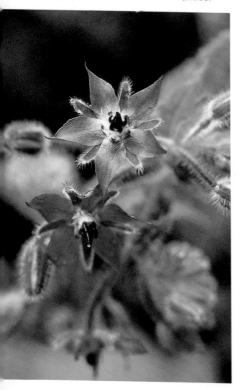

▾ *The delicate star-shaped flowers of the borage plant can be eaten raw in salads.*

herbal cough linctus

25g/1oz fresh or 15g/½oz dried thyme
25g/1oz fresh or 15g/½oz dried
    borage flowers and leaves
2 x 5cm/2in cinnamon sticks
600ml/1 pint/2½ cups water
juice of 1 small lemon
100g/4oz/½ cup honey

Put the herbs into a non-aluminium pan with the cinnamon and water. Bring to the boil, cover and simmer for 20 minutes. Strain off the liquid and return to the pan. Simmer, uncovered, until the liquid is reduced by half. Stir in the lemon juice and honey and simmer gently for 5 minutes. Pour into a screw-top bottle and refrigerate.

The cooling and cleansing properties of borage make it useful for detoxifying the system and for any condition associated with excess heat.

26 thyme & sage gargle

Regular use of mouthwashes and gargles helps keep the mouth and throat germ-free. At the onset of a cold, gargle with an infusion of sage and thyme to ease the discomfort of a sore throat.

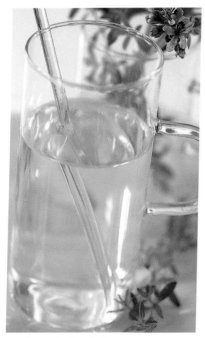

▲ *Thyme fortifies the immune system in its fight against bacterial and viral infections.*

Both thyme and sage are powerful antiseptics, sage having a particular affinity with the mouth and throat, and thyme with the chest and lungs. The two herbs together make a powerful combination for treating the symptoms of a cold, particularly sore throats and tickly coughs. If you are able to catch the symptoms quickly enough you may be able to prevent them from developing.

Making your own gargle or cough medicine is quick and easy using an infusion of fresh or dried herbs. Gargle with the mix three or four times a day, or take 10ml/2 tsp, three or four times a day as a soothing linctus.

sore throat gargle

small handful of fresh sage flowers and leaves or 30ml/2 tbsp dried herb
small handful of thyme flowers and leaves or 30ml/2 tbsp dried herb
600ml/1 pint/2½ cups boiling water
30ml/2 tbsp cider vinegar
10ml/2 tsp honey
5ml/1 tsp cayenne pepper

Place the fresh or dried herbs into a jug, pour in the boiling water, cover and leave to infuse for 30 minutes. Strain off the water and stir in the cider vinegar, honey and cayenne. Pour the mixture into a screw-top bottle and keep in a cool place. The mixture will keep for 1 week.

27 garlic & honey syrup

The compounds contained in garlic can help prevent
and cure infection. Garlic is one of the most powerful
natural remedies for treating coughs, colds and flu.
Use it with honey to make a soothing cold cure.

Garlic has powerful antiseptic and
antiviral properties and combines
well with honey, which is soothing,
to make a syrup to prevent or
relieve cold and flu symptoms. Take
15ml/1 tbsp three times a day as a
preventative, or to ease the first signs
of a cold. The syrup will keep for up
to 2-3 weeks in the refrigerator.

garlic cold cure
1 head of garlic
300ml/½ pint/1¼ cups water
juice of ½ lemon
30ml/2 tbsp honey

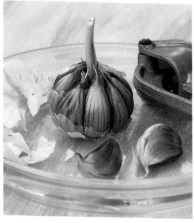

▲ Use garlic to ward off colds and flu.

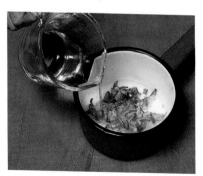

1 Wash and crush the garlic cloves –
there is no need to peel them. Put them
in a pan with the water. Bring to the boil,
cover and simmer gently for 20 minutes.

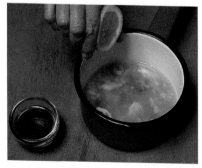

2 Add the lemon juice and honey and
simmer for 2-3 minutes. Let the mixture
cool, then strain it into a clean, dark
glass jar or bottle with an airtight lid.

28 marshmallow soother

If left untreated, a heavy cold can turn into more serious health problems such as laryngitis or bronchitis. Use marshmallow to treat an acute sore throat, hoarseness and a dry, hacking cough.

The name of the marshmallow plant is derived from a Greek word meaning "to heal" and the plant is well known for its ability to soothe and heal bronchial disorders. The heart-shaped leaves and the soft pink flowers have a protective and soothing action on the mucus membranes: they both encourage the expulsion of phlegm and can relieve dry coughs, bronchial asthma, bronchial catarrh and pleurisy.

The following gargle combines marshmallow with cider vinegar, also known for its antiseptic and healing properties, and should help relieve a painful throat and dry, hacking cough. Use it three or four times a day, or take it as a linctus: 10ml/2 tsp, two or three times a day.

marshmallow gargle
1 small handful of fresh marshmallow or 30ml/2 tbsp of the dried herb
600ml/1 pint/2½ cups boiling water
30ml/2 tbsp cider vinegar
30ml/2 tbsp honey

Add the fresh or dried marshmallow to a jug containing the boiling water. Cover and leave to infuse for up to

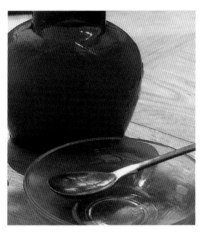

▲ Herbal remedies keep best in a dark glass bottle or jar with a tight-fitting lid.

30 minutes and then strain off the herbs. Stir in the cider vinegar and the honey to taste. Pour the mixture into a dark bottle or jar with a screw-top lid. It will keep for up to 1 week stored in a cool place.

Infections of the upper respiratory tract should be taken seriously and treated as soon as possible. If they do not respond to home treatment, seek medical advice.

29 lavender balm

A sore, red nose, dry lips and cold sores often accompany a cold. These symptoms are best treated locally by the application of a soothing skin salve containing healing plant oils.

Beeswax and cocoa butter form a good basis for a salve. They are rich emollients and will help to moisturize the skin. Wheatgerm oil is high in vitamin E, and seems to work wonders when applied to dry skin. It also helps to preserve the cream.

Lavender is a good addition to a skin salve as it has antiseptic, antiviral and anti-inflammatory properties. Its antiviral properties are particularly useful for treating cold sores. The best way of using it in a cream is to add a few drops of the essential oil.

▾ *Lavender promotes the rapid healing of broken skin and soothes inflammation.*

lavender skin soother
5ml/1 tsp beeswax
5ml/1 tsp cocoa butter
5ml/1 tsp wheatgerm oil
5ml/1 tsp almond oil

Add the ingredients to a small bowl. Set the bowl over a pan of simmering water and stir the contents until the wax has melted.

Remove the bowl from the heat and allow the mixture to cool for a few minutes before adding 3 drops of lavender essential oil. Pour the mix into a small, screw-topped jar and leave to set. Store the cream away from the light and use as required.

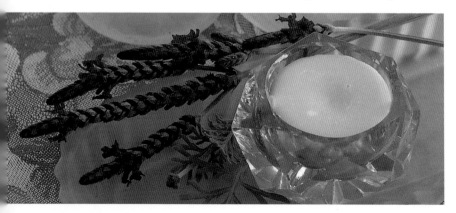

30

lavender & eucalyptus rub

A blocked nose is one of the most miserable aspects of having a cold. An old-fashioned back and chest rub with lavender and eucalyptus can work wonders to ease sinus congestion.

Lavender and eucalyptus used together make an effective decongestant rub. Eucalyptus is a traditional Aboriginal fever remedy, and the essential oil is one of the most antiseptic of herbal essences. The oil's aroma is both penetrating and refreshing, and an immune-system stimulant. Lavender also has powerful antiseptic and antibiotic properties, and a decongesting and expectorant action. It is also an effective sedative.

bedtime chest rub
50g/2oz petroleum jelly
15ml/1 tbsp dried lavender heads
6 drops eucalyptus essential oil
4 drops camphor essential oil

Melt the petroleum jelly in a bowl over a pan of simmering water. Stir in the lavender and heat for 30 minutes. Strain the liquid jelly through a piece of muslin and allow to cool before adding the essential oils. Pour the mix into a clean jar and leave until set.

Massage the rub on to the throat, chest and upper back at bedtime so the oils penetrate the skin and the vapours are inhaled throughout the night.

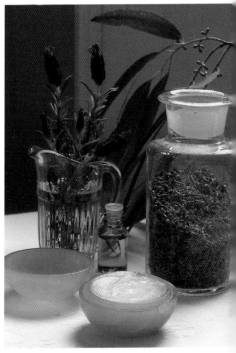

▲ Use fresh or dried lavender heads and eucalyptus oil in a chest and back rub.

CAUTION
Eucalyptus and camphor should be avoided if taking homeopathic treatment.

31 herbal compresses

Natural medicine sees fever as an important healing process. Herbal extracts can be applied to the body on hot or cold compresses to help bring the fever out and/or down.

Compresses are made by making a herbal infusion and then soaking a clean cloth in the hot water. The cloth is then wrung out and either applied to the body while it is still warm or left to cool before applying.

hot compress
Chamomile, cypress, juniper, lavender, peppermint, tea tree and rosemary will all induce sweating if the body needs to sweat. Drop a handful of fresh or dried herbs into a basin of hot water and leave to infuse for 5-10 minutes. Soak a clean cloth in the water, wring it out and use while hand-hot as needed.

cold compress
Bergamot, eucalyptus, lavender and peppermint have a cooling effect on the body and are useful to bring a fever down when it is dangerously high. Again, make an infusion with a handful of fresh or dried herbs dropped into a basin of hot water and leave to infuse as before. Let the water cool before soaking a clean cloth in it. Wring out the cloth and apply to the forehead or the back of the neck.

Lavender and peppermint have a balancing action on the body and can be used for both hot and cold compresses.

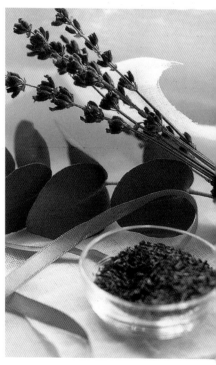

▲ *Eucalyptus and lavender are effective on a cool compress to bring a fever down.*

32 elderflower tincture

Tinctures have a reasonably long shelf-life and are an effective way to extract the active ingredients of plants. They can be made with fresh or dried plant material steeped in a mixture of alcohol and water.

The creamy white blossoms of the elder tree are an excellent remedy for the onset of colds and flu. At the first signs of discomfort – aching, sore throat, chills, restlessness and fever – elderflowers will stimulate the system and cause sweating. Sweating cleanses the body, eliminating toxins via the pores of the skin, and is the body's way of throwing off infection. Elderflowers also have a relaxing and decongestant action on the bronchi, reducing muscle spasm and also helping to expel any phlegm.

You can benefit from the healing properties of elderflowers all the year round by making them into a tincture. Preserved in an alcohol base, the tincture will keep for up to 2 years. Since tinctures are highly concentrated extracts, you should not exceed a dosage of more than 5ml/ 1 tsp, three or four times a day. You can dilute your elderflower tincture in a little water or add to your favourite fruit juice if preferred.

▸ *The anticatarrhal properties of elder tree blossoms make them an excellent choice for making a cold-cure tincture.*

cold-cure tincture

15g/½ oz dried elderflowers
250ml/8fl oz/1 cup vodka
made up to 300ml/½ pint/1¼ cups with water

Put the dried elderflowers into a glass jar and pour in the vodka and water mixture. Seal the jar and leave in a cool, dark place for 7-10 days (no longer), shaking occasionally. Strain off the elderflowers through a sieve lined with kitchen paper before pouring the mixture into a sterilized bottle. Store in a cool, dark place.

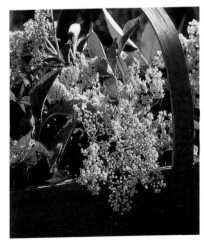

33 rose petal tonic

Rose leaves and petals have a cooling effect, which is useful for bringing down a fever and clearing heat and toxins from the body. Preserve their healing properties in a medicinal vinegar.

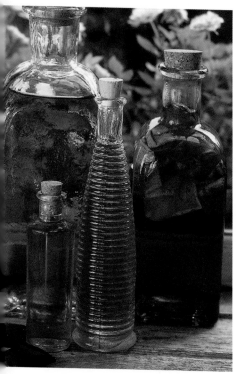

▲ *Rose petal vinegar is a tonic for a cold.*

Raspberry vinegar, made with 115g/4oz raspberries and 600ml/ 1 pint/2½ cups cider vinegar is useful for treating sore throats.

Cider vinegar is the preferred choice for making a medicinal vinegar. It is an antiseptic and has a balancing action on the body. Dried or fresh rose leaves and petals are then added to the vinegar and left to steep.

The soothing, astringent action of rose petals is strengthening to the lungs and is useful for relieving cold and flu symptoms, easing a sore throat and drying up a runny nose. Rose also has an uplifting effect on the spirits and can ease a headache.

rose petal vinegar
50g/2oz fresh rose petals
600ml/1 pint/2½ cups cider vinegar

For a soothing rose vinegar, put the ingredients in a screw-top jar. Screw on the lid and leave in a warm place for 10 days. Strain off the liquid into a sterilized seal-top container and store in a cool, dark place.

The vinegar may be used as a gargle for the throat or taken as a linctus: 5ml/1 tsp, three or four times a day. Alternatively, dab a few drops on to a tissue and apply to the temples to ease a feverish headache.

34 four thieves cold cure

This traditional recipe is attributed to a gang of four thieves who avoided catching the plague in medieval France by making liberal use of a strong herbal vinegar. Try it to guard against colds and flu.

Many versions of the recipe have been attributed to the four thieves. This formula, based on an amalgam of the old recipes, is effective as a mild antiseptic, or to take in prophylactic doses of 5ml/1 tsp, two or three times a day, when exposed to colds and other viral infections. The recipe benefits from the health-giving properties of cider vinegar.

four thieves vinegar
15ml/1 tbsp each dried lavender,
   rosemary, sage and peppermint
2–3 bay leaves
10ml/2 tsp dried wormwood
5ml/1 tsp garlic granules
5ml/1 tsp ground cloves

5ml/1 tsp ground cinnamon
600ml/1 pint/2½ cups cider vinegar
Put all the dry ingredients into a jar and fill it with the cider vinegar. Cover tightly and leave in a warm place, such as on a sunny windowsill or by a central heating boiler, for 10 days. Strain off the liquid, through a sieve lined with kitchen paper, into a clean jug. Finally, pour the vinegar into a sterilized bottle and seal.

▼ *Ingredients for Four Thieves Vinegar (clockwise from right): lavender and bay, rosemary, peppermint, cloves, cinnamon and wormwood, garlic and sage.*

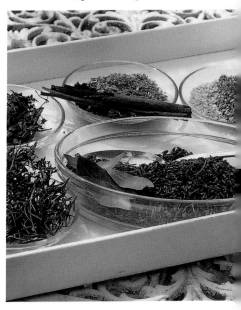

CAUTIONS
• Do not take internally for more than 2 weeks at a time.

• Do not take if pregnant, as wormwood is a uterine stimulant.

35 fresh herb inhalant

For centuries, steam inhalations have been used to ease problems in the respiratory tract, including coughs, colds, sinus congestion and sore throats. Hundreds of herbs are suitable for this purpose.

To make a steam inhalant, the most usual method is to add boiling water to a bowl of freshly picked herbs and/or spices. For a congested cold, try the effective recipe opposite.

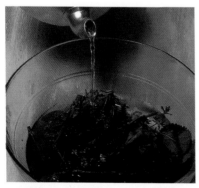

▲ Pour boiling water into a bowl of fresh herbs and some spices.

CAUTION
Inhalations should be carefully monitored if the person is asthmatic or suffers from hay fever or any allergy. If this is the case, they should only be used for up to 1 minute; providing this provokes no adverse reaction, the time can gradually be increased up to 3-5 minutes.

cold decongester
Select a handful of herbs and/or spices from the following: eucalyptus leaves, basil, hyssop, juniper foliage and berries, lavender, lemon balm, mint, rosemary, sage, thyme, cayenne pepper, and cinnamon sticks. All of these herbs and spices have a detoxifying effect and will help to clear the airways.

Put the selected herbs and spices into a bowl. Pour in about 1 litre/1¾ pints/ 4 cups of boiling water. Lean over the bowl, covering it and your head with a towel. Sit in the steam and inhale the herbal aromas for 5-10 minutes, or as long as is comfortable.

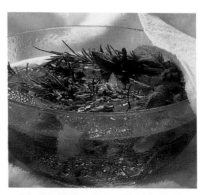

▲ Inhaling the fragrance of fresh herbs is a satisfying way to clear the nasal passages.

36 mustard foot bath

Taking a foot bath can restore and revitalize the whole body. Add mustard for a relaxing and therapeutic experience that will help combat the symptoms of a head cold or feverish chill.

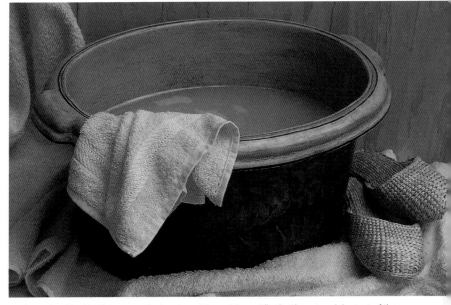

▲ *A mustard foot bath is a popular treatment for colds and flu that has stood the test of time.*

Black mustard is a well-known spice. Its main therapeutic use is as an external application. Mustard has a warming, stimulating effect on the circulation, encouraging sweating and relieving muscular aches and pains. At the onset of a cold or chill, a mustard foot bath will have a warming and comforting effect.

warming foot bath
Pour 2.2 litres/4 pints/9 cups hot water into a large bowl. Add 15ml/1 tbsp mustard powder to the water and stir it well until it is dissolved. Immerse the feet while the bath is still hot and sit back and relax for 20-30 minutes. Keep topping up the bowl with hot water if necessary.

37

essential oils

Essential oils capture the essence of the plant and all its healing properties in a highly concentrated form. Aromatherapy describes the use of these oils for therapeutic purposes.

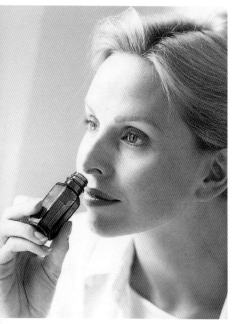

▲ *Inhaling an essential oil is a quick way of enjoying its health-giving properties.*

Aromatherapy works by inhalation and/or by absorption into the skin. With one or two exceptions, oils are never put directly on to the skin but are added to a suitable carrier base, such as water (for bathing) or vegetable oil (for massage).

aromatherapy cold cures

There are many essential oils that can be comforting and helpful for a cold. Some of the most effective include tea tree and eucalyptus, which have a long tradition of use in Aboriginal medicine. Both oils are powerful antiseptics with a clean and penetrating "medicinal" aroma.

Peppermint, rosemary, lavender, frankincense, sandalwood and jasmine are also useful for a cold. Peppermint and rosemary have a fresh, uplifting aroma, which can help to clear blocked sinuses and relieve a stuffy head cold. Lavender is an antiviral and an immunity booster; it also soothes inflammation and restores balance to the body.

Frankincense and sandalwood are especially good for easing congestion in chesty coughs and colds, and jasmine oil is also useful for treating catarrh and chest infections.

CAUTION

Essential oils are not for internal use and should be handled with care and respect.

38 aromatic inhalations

A steam inhalation warms and moistens the airways. Adding essential oils helps to open and relax the airways, clearing the congested nasal passages and soothing the mucous membranes.

To make the most out of a steam inhalation, have the steam as hot as possible, without actually burning the nose and throat. Very hot steam is in itself a hostile environment for viruses and works well with the antibacterial and antiviral action of the oils to kill off many germs.

For an inhalation to relieve a stuffy head cold, a combination of eucalyptus and tea tree oil is ideal. Studies show that tea tree oil is active against all types of infectious organisms: bacteria, fungi and viruses. It is also a very powerful immune stimulant, increasing the body's ability to respond to these organisms. Eucalyptus also has a powerful antibacterial and antiviral action, and its sharply penetrating aroma is well known as a decongestant.

eucalyptus and tea tree inhalation
Boil a kettle and pour approximately 600ml/1 pint/2½ cups hot water into a large bowl – one the size of a washing-up bowl is ideal. Add 3 drops of tea tree and 2 drops of eucalyptus. Sit in front of the bowl with a towel draped over your head and shoulders to form a tent. As the oils vaporize, breathe in the steam as deeply as possible. The action of the oils should begin to decongest blocked nasal passages, kill off the germs and soothe the unpleasant cold symptoms.

If you prefer, rosemary and peppermint oils may be substituted to achieve a similar result.

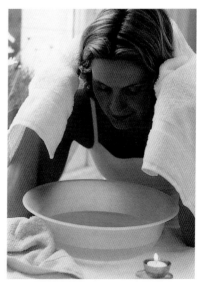

▲ Inhaling steam scented with eucalyptus or tea tree oil is a powerful antiseptic that will help to decongest blocked sinuses.

39 cold-treatment massage

The power of touch to comfort and bring healing to the body is widely recognized. Essential oils can be used in an upper back and chest massage to make a relaxing and effective cold treatment.

Massage is not only relaxing and a good tension-easer, it also boosts the immune system and helps the body to eliminate toxins. When using essential oils in massage, they must be added to a suitable massage oil or unperfumed cream/lotion base. High-quality vegetable oils, such as sunflower, almond or wheatgerm, are

ideal as a massage base oil. Use a total of 4-5 drops of essential oil to 30ml/ 2 tbsp base oil, lotion or cream.

selecting an essential oil

There are many essential oils that can help a cold, particularly tea tree, peppermint, lavender and eucalyptus. Additionally, marjoram can ease a tickly cough and chest congestion, and myrrh is also helpful for thick catarrh and a whooping-type cough. If the cold has given way to laryngitis, try a combination of sandalwood, niaouli and lemon grass oils massaged on to the upper back and chest.

upper back and chest massage

To give the massage, gently spread the oil across the upper back and chest and work it into the skin. On the back, this can be done with a wide stroking movement, on the front use small circular movements with the tips of the fingers. Notice any areas that feel particularly tight or tender and give them an extra working. If you don't have anyone to give you a back massage, the treatment is equally effective as an upper chest rub.

▾ *Massage stimulates the circulation and encourages the elimination of toxins.*

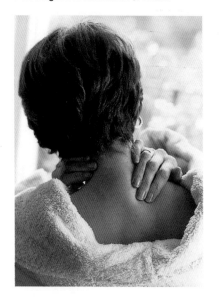

40 facial massage

Almost any part of the body benefits from being massaged. To ease sinus congestion, a gentle facial self-massage will encourage drainage of mucus from the nose and sinuses.

The massage can be done with or without essential oils. Select the oils according to your symptoms. If there is a dull pain in the forehead and sinus cavities, lavender and thyme are effective, whereas tea tree, eucalyptus, peppermint and pine are all good at clearing congestion. Add 4–5 drops of the combined essential oils to 30ml/2 tbsp of massage oil. The following routine is best done after an aromatic steam inhalation, which will have opened up the airways and softened the mucus.

sinus self-massage

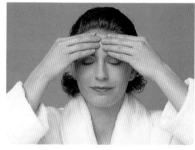

1 Start all over your brow, beginning at the centre and working out with small circular motions from your fingertips.

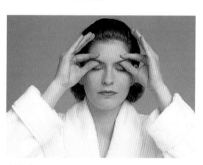

2 Release pressure from the sinus passages by pinching along the ridge of your eyebrows with your thumbs and index fingers, starting on the inside corners and working, step by step, to the outer edge.

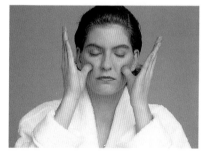

3 The small indentations beneath the ridges of the cheekbones indicate the site of some of the sinus passages. Apply thumb pressure slowly up into the hollows. Hold for a count of five and release. This will help to clear the head.

41 essential oil bath

Bathing with essential oils is one of the simplest and yet most effective aromatherapy treatments. An aromatic bath can help to detoxify the body and ease the symptoms of colds and viral infections.

Essential oils have a dual action in the bath: they are absorbed through the skin into the bloodstream, while their aromas are inhaled, working directly on the senses and emotions.

baths for a cold
There are many different oils that are suitable for treating coughs, colds and flu. Fill the bath first with comfortably hot water then add the essential oil/s

▼ *Pamper yourself with an aromatic bath.*

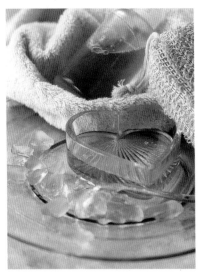

just before you get in, swirling the water round to disperse them. To avoid an oily scum around the bath, you can mix them together first in a little milk or add them to an unscented foam bubble bath.

- At the first sign of a cold, bathing with tea tree oil can often stop the cold developing. Run a hot bath and swish 2-3 drops of the oil to the water.

- For a cold with a cough, a combination of rosemary, sage and peppermint will make an energizing morning bath. Add 1 drop of each oil to the water.

- A fluey cold will benefit from a rosemary, peppermint and ginger mix. Add 1 drop of each oil to a morning bath.

- When convalescing after a heavy cold, enjoy a relaxing evening bath with 2 drops of lavender, 1 drop rose and 1 drop ylang ylang oil.

42

hand & foot baths

In the shivery, aching, hot-and-cold stage of a feverish cold or flu, a hand or foot bath may be a better option than a full-body bath. Add essential oils of ginger and nutmeg to warm the body.

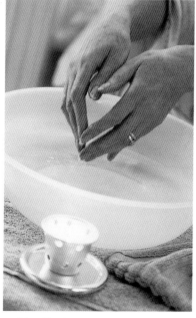

▲ A hand bath using a blend of ginger and nutmeg oil will help ease a fluey cold.

The essential oils of nutmeg and ginger are useful for treating a shivery, runny-nosed winter cold. Similar to cinnamon, nutmeg oil has a stimulating effect on the body, helping to warm and tone it up and build resistance to colds. Ginger is also a stimulating, warming oil and useful for colds. Similar to the fresh root, its fiery properties are useful for treating any condition associated with excess damp; it heats up the body and helps to dry out excess moisture.

winter warmer

To make a hand or foot bath, fill a large bowl two-thirds full with hot water. Add 1 drop of each essential oil and swish the water before sitting back with your hands or feet in the bowl. Give yourself a soak for 10-15 minutes. The warmth of the water will help the blood vessels to dilate and the body to relax, while the oils are absorbed into the bloodstream.

CAUTIONS
• Ginger and nutmeg oils should be used with care as they may cause a skin reaction in some individuals. If in doubt, do a skin-patch test first on the inside of the wrist or elbow.

• Do not use nutmeg oil if you are pregnant or breastfeeding.

Add a few drops of **lavender oil** to a cool **compress** to **ease** aching limbs and a hot, burning headache.

44 homeopathy

Homeopathy views symptoms as the body's attempt to heal itself. A homeopathic remedy is selected on the basis of a "picture" of these symptoms, which will vary between individuals.

Most homeopathic remedies are prepared from a tincture of an original plant or mineral substance. This is then diluted many times, until barely a trace of the original substance remains. Instead, the remedy is thought to contain an "energy blueprint" of the original substance, which then works on the body's energy system, to stimulate the self-healing process.

selecting a cold remedy

As homeopathic treatment is unique to the individual, choose the remedy that best fits with your "symptom-picture". Take three times a day in the 6C potency or once a day in the 30C potency until symptoms improve.

▾ *Homeopathic remedies are available as a small, tasteless pill, or as drops.*

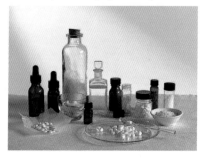

ACONITE: symptoms that come on suddenly, often at night. Flu is marked by profuse sweating and a high fever.

ALLIUM CEPA or *ARSENICUM*: at the first sign of a head cold, try either of these two remedies. Allium cepa is marked by watery eyes and a runny nose, and Arsenicum by looking pale and feeling chilly.

BELLADONNA: symptoms that come on quickly with a high fever, marked by redness, burning heat and a throbbing headache.

BRYONIA: symptoms come on more slowly, accompanied by extreme thirst, irritability and the desire to be left alone.

GELSEMIUM: this is the most widely used flu remedy. The most pronounced symptoms are shaking with shivering, aching muscles and general weakness.

FERRUM PHOS: for symptoms that are not well defined or as a general tonic during and after the flu.

45 reiki healing

Reiki is a Japanese healing system based on channelling healing energy to the body. Receiving reiki is a relaxing experience and can help with common ailments such as coughs and colds.

Reiki healing can bring rapid relief from a common cold; the subtle healing energy is so effective, that symptoms have been known to clear up almost instantaneously. Reiki works by putting the hands in certain positions on the body and then allowing the healing energy to flow through them.

Reiki is learned by being initiated or "attuned" by a Reiki Master. Reiki classes are widely available.

reiki cold treatment

To give a reiki treatment, stand to one side of the recipient and place one hand on the forehead and your other hand on the centre of the chest. This will help relieve a headache, an aching neck and shoulders, blocked airways and coughing. The position of the hand on the chest is also comforting and relaxing.

Leave the hands in this position until you feel it's enough. Then move to stand behind the recipient and place the fingers of both hands under the cheekbones. This will help to ease congestion in the sinuses.

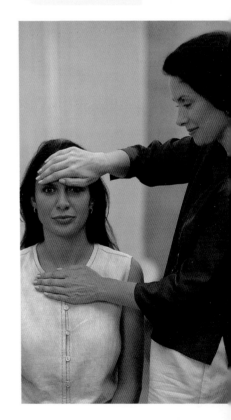

▸ *A reiki treatment can have many therapeutic and healing benefits for both the practitioner and the receiver.*

46 reflexology massage

By applying gentle pressure to certain points on the feet, reflexology stimulates the body to heal itself. Reflexology can boost the immune system and treat colds, sore throats and sinus problems.

Reflex zones on the hands or feet correspond to different organs of the body via energy paths, or meridians. To treat a cold with blocked or painful sinuses, you need to give all the toes a good working as this is where the sinus reflexes are situated. The large area beneath them on the underside of the feet corresponds to the chest.

After a treatment it is a good idea to relax and keep yourself warm. It is also important to drink plenty of water to help the body flush out the toxins released during the treatment.

cold treatment routine

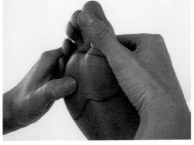

1 Begin by working the whole chest area. This will help the airways open up and encourage clear breathing.

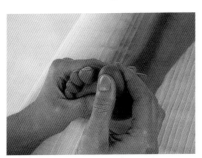

2 Beginning with the big toe, apply firm pressure to the tops of all the toes. This will help to clear the sinuses. Then pinpoint the pituitary gland in the centre of the prints of both big toes to stimulate the endocrine system.

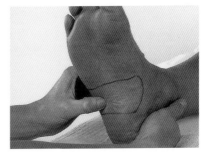

3 Treat the upper lymph system by working down the front of the toes to stimulate the immune system. Then work the large area above the heel to stimulate the small intestines and colon. This helps the body to eliminate toxins.

47 colour meditation

Tap into the power of the mind to bring healing and wellbeing to the body. Use meditation and creative visualization to encourage a speedy recovery from colds and other common complaints.

This healing meditation is best done sitting or lying down somewhere warm and quiet where you will not be disturbed for around 15-20 minutes. The meditation can be practised at any time of the day, or last thing at night to promote a restful sleep.

healing with colour

Begin by imagining a healing glow of coloured light surrounding your body. Let that colour become stronger and then as you breathe in, imagine it flowing into the top of your head. As you continue to relax, let the coloured light begin to suffuse all areas of your body, starting with the head, face, neck and shoulders, and travel down, penetrating all the muscles and organs. Fill up every part of your body until it is completely suffused with a warm, healing light.

As you relax, bring your attention to the head, throat and chest area, or any other area of the body you feel drawn to. Draw in more warmth and colour on the in-breath and send it to this area. Imagine it giving power, helping to strengthen the cells and

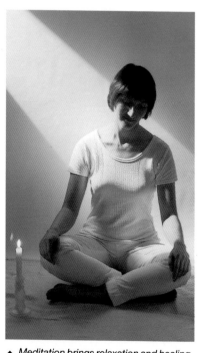

▲ *Meditation brings relaxation and healing.*

fight off germs. Imagine your body free of aches and pains and any illness.

When you feel the healing is complete, allow the light to disperse, letting it go with each exhalation. Gently stretch your body as you return to the everyday world.

48 amethyst healing

Crystals and stones are used in healing to magnify and transform energy. Amethyst quartz is one of the most useful healing stones. Its cleansing and balancing properties can be used to treat a cold.

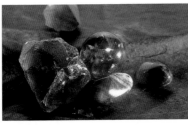

◀ Amethyst quartz is one of the most versatile healing stones.

Many healers believe that illness originates in the body's subtle energy system of chakras and auras. Crystals can be used to help realign these energies and bring about healing.

For a cold that lingers on and won't seem to shift, you could try treating it on another level, using amethyst points to rebalance and repair any "holes" in the aura.

crystal cold cure

Make sure you can lie somewhere warm and quiet for 20-30 minutes, where you won't be disturbed. You may like to play a piece of soothing music during the relaxation. Take eight amethysts of roughly equal size, and space them out evenly around the body. If the stones are faceted, place them so that the points are facing inwards; this will focus the healing energy towards the body. Now lie back and relax as the stones realign your aura.

▼ Amethyst balances and quietens the mind.

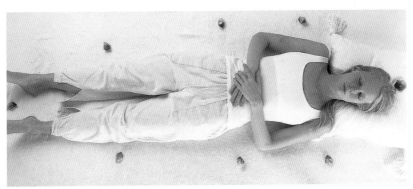

49

go to bed

Sleep is probably one of the greatest natural healers of all. Sometimes the body just needs a chance to rest and recuperate from the stresses and strains of daily life.

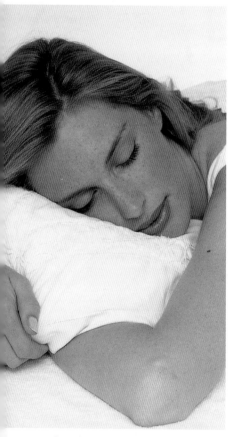

When you have a cold or flu, make sure you have plenty of rest and sleep – this alone will go a long way towards a quick recovery. Always make sure you sleep in a well-ventilated room. It is better to put an extra blanket on the bed and sleep with the window slightly open than to spend the night in a stuffy, overheated room.

▼ *A lavender sachet beside the bed may help to induce sleep.*

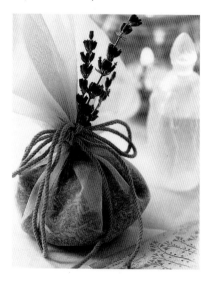

▲ *One of the best cures for a cold is to make yourself a herb or spice tea and go straight to bed.*

Try resting your head on a
sleep pillow
filled with mild sedative
herbs and flowers such as
hops or
lavender.

index

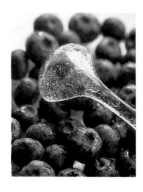

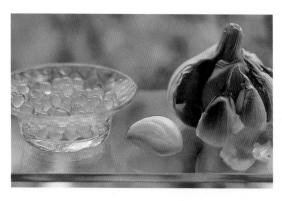

index

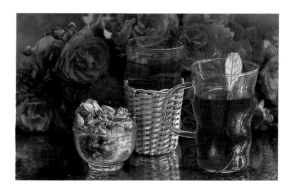

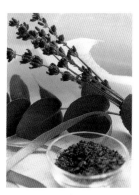

This edition is published by Lorenz Books,
an imprint of Anness Publishing Ltd,
Blaby Road, Wigston, Leicestershire LE18 4SE; info@anness.com

www.lorenzbooks.com; www.annesspublishing.com

If you like the images in this book and would like to investigate using them for
publishing, promotions or advertising, please visit our website
www.practicalpictures.com for more information.

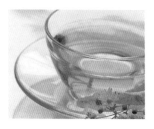

A CIP catalogue record for this book is available from the British Library.

Publisher: Joanna Lorenz
Managing editor: Helen Sudell
Editor: Melanie Halton
Design: Jester Designs
Production Manager: Steve Lang
Editorial reader: Jonathan Marshall
Indexer: Hilary Bird

Publisher's note:
The reader should not regard the recommendations, ideas and techniques expressed
and described in this book as substitutes for the advice of a qualified medical
practitioner or other qualified professional. Any use to which the recommendations,
ideas and techniques are put is at the reader's sole discretion and risk.

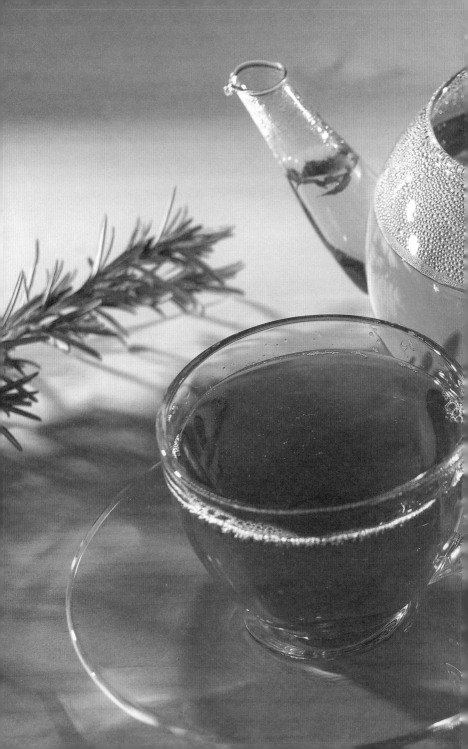